1 MONTH OF
FREE
READING

at

www.ForgottenBooks.com

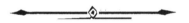

By purchasing this book you are eligible for one month membership to ForgottenBooks.com, giving you unlimited access to our entire collection of over 1,000,000 titles via our web site and mobile apps.

To claim your free month visit:

www.forgottenbooks.com/free559704

ISBN 978-0-483-95873-9
PIBN 10559704

stitutes for the natural teeth when these have been lost, they are not like the teeth which nature makes. In a sense they are comparable to the artificial contrivances with which we replace natural limbs. They are an added care. In many mouths it is not possible to give them a good fixation; and their efficiency in mastication is much less than that of natural teeth.

An important circumstance with reference to the possession of good teeth is hereditary influence. The laws of transmission from parent to child which obtain in other particulars exercise their influence upon the characteristics of the teeth. Children that are born of parents with poor, soft, rapidly-decaying teeth are likely to inherit similar dental peculiarities. Conversely, children born of good parentage, whose teeth have been regular, little inclined to decay, and generally strong, are likely to possess teeth resembling those of their parents.

Next after the matter of heredity are the circumstances surrounding the early life of the child. This is true with reference to the child's entire environment, — its home life, its fresh air, its outdoor exercise, its sleep, and especially its diet. If these particulars of the home life are wisely controlled, the teeth of the children share in the benefits. If there is ignorance and a lack of proper regard for these things, and especially if such ignorance is added to a bad heredity, it is only natural that we should find, as we do find, that the teeth of the children are poor, soft, inclined to decay and apt to be lost early.

I had these facts forcibly impressed upon me through having been for a time in my early studies in dentistry in a manufacturing city in Massachusetts, having a population including many not of the most favored class. A great number of the parents were of foreign birth, and the ancestry of the children was often mixed. The homes in which they

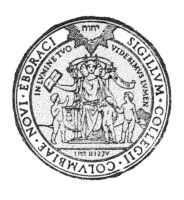

HARVARD HEALTH TALKS

THE CARE AND FEEDING OF
CHILDREN
BY JOHN LOVETT MORSE

PRESERVATIVES AND OTHER
CHEMICALS IN FOODS: THEIR USE
AND ABUSE
BY OTTO FOLIN

THE CARE OF THE SKIN
BY CHARLES JAMES WHITE

THE CARE OF THE SICK ROOM
BY ELBRIDGE GERRY CUTLER

THE CARE OF THE TEETH
BY CHARLES ALBERT BRACKETT

HARVARD HEALTH TALKS

HARVARD HEALTH TALKS

THE CARE OF THE TEETH

BY

CHARLES A. BRACKETT, D.M.D.

PROFESSOR OF DENTAL PATHOLOGY IN
HARVARD UNIVERSITY

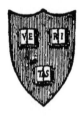

CAMBRIDGE
HARVARD UNIVERSITY PRESS
1915

HARVARD HEALTH TALKS

PRESENTING the substance of some of the public lectures delivered at the Medical School of Harvard University, this series aims to provide in easily accessible form modern and authoritative information on medical subjects of general importance. The following committee, composed of members of the Faculty of Medicine, has editorial supervision of the volumes published:

EDWARD HICKLING BRADFORD, A.M., M.D., Dean of the Faculty of Medicine, and Professor of Orthopedic Surgery, Emeritus.

HAROLD CLARENCE ERNST, A.M., M.D., Professor of Bacteriology.

WALTER BRADFORD CANNON, A.M., M.D., George Higginson Professor of Physiology.

THE CARE OF THE TEETH

THE CARE OF THE TEETH

THE importance of this subject needs no argument. Symmetrical, sound, well-kept teeth are important contributions to the beauty of the human countenance. Their possession is rightly construed to mean cultivation and refinement. A person with nicely kept teeth may be expected to be of the kind fastidious in other particulars. Then in addition to the beauty of the teeth, may be urged their importance in the preparation of the food for digestion and assimilation. All other things being equal, the person who masticates his food thoroughly is the person likely to be blessed with the most comfortable and complete digestion, and the best nutrition.

While it is true that the prosthetic dentist is able to provide excellent substitutes for the natural teeth when these have been lost, they are not like the teeth which nature makes. In a sense they are comparable to the artificial contrivances with which we replace natural limbs. They are an added care. In many mouths it is not possible to give them a good fixation; and their efficiency in mastication is much less than that of natural teeth.

An important circumstance with reference to the possession of good teeth is hereditary influence. The laws of transmission from parent to child which obtain in other particulars exercise their influence upon the characteristics of the teeth. Children that are born of parents with poor, soft, rapidly-decaying teeth are likely to inherit similar dental peculiarities. Conversely, children born of good parentage, whose teeth have been regular, little inclined to decay, and generally strong, are likely to possess teeth resembling those of their parents.

CARE OF THE TEETH

Next after the matter of heredity are the circumstances surrounding the early life of the child. This is true with reference to the child's entire environment, — its home life, its fresh air, its outdoor exercise, its sleep, and especially its diet. If these particulars of the home life are wisely controlled, the teeth of the children share in the benefits. If there is ignorance and a lack of proper regard for these things, and especially if such ignorance is added to a bad heredity, it is only natural that we should find, as we do find, that the teeth of the children are poor, soft, inclined to decay and apt to be lost early.

I had these facts forcibly impressed upon me through having been for a time in my early studies in dentistry in a manufacturing city in Massachusetts, having a population including many not of the most favored class. A great number of the parents were of foreign birth, and the ancestry of the children was often mixed. The homes in which they lived, and the general circumstances of their lives, were unfavorable. A considerable portion of their diet was made up of a poor quality of baker's bread and molasses, a combination not only lacking in nutritional elements important for the teeth, but also readily fermentable; and the products of this fermentation are especially harmful to the teeth, as we shall see a little later. Among those children, I have many times seen the teeth of the temporary set at the age of four years little more than a mass of decaying roots in suppurating gums, — a deplorable condition, in every particular, for the child's well-being.

From this manufacturing city I went to begin the practice of dentistry in the place which has since been my home, — a residential city including, particularly in the summer, many who possess in large measure what are usually called the advantages of life. In this community I came immediately and directly in contact with a class of people diametrically opposite to that which I have just described. They were people whose stock was vouched for by that distinguished success in life which gave them their accumulated large means, with its associated cultivation. In these families the homes of the children, the regimen under which they were brought up, the food which they had, the fresh air, outdoor exercise and the abundance of sleep which were provided for them, had their legitimate consequences in a quality of teeth and a health of mouth the very opposite of those which I had seen in the other city. The result, in each instance, was but the natural consequence of the operation of influential causes.

Perhaps I can best speak next of the care of children's teeth, of the reasons why children's teeth should have good care, and of how that care should be given.

It is essential for a child's well-being that its first teeth be in a state of comfort and serviceableness, and that they be retained in their places until the permanent teeth are ready to succeed them. If a child has open, sensitive cavities in its teeth, they are a source of suffering, of discomfort and incapacity in chewing; and if these cavities are permitted to progress until there are exposed pulps, there is ordinarily pain, from which the child may suffer extremely, and which, especially when occurring at night, will be a marked source of disquietude in the family. Then if the child, on account of neglect of its teeth, and the development of penetrating caries with its associated pain, prematurely loses teeth, especially any of the back teeth of the temporary set, there is very likely to be irregularity in the permanent set as a result.

The teeth of the child, the temporary teeth, are ordinarily in their place at the age of three years. Contrary to the ideas generally held among parents, none of these teeth fall out until nature has brought into their places the four largest and strongest teeth of the permanent set.

The child's set of teeth is twenty in number, ten in each jaw, five in each quarter of the mouth. The first teeth of the permanent set to appear are almost invariably in place, in a position immediately behind the farthest back teeth of the child's set, at the age of six years. These established, nature replaces one of the five temporary teeth in each quarter of the mouth each year in this order: — the central incisor at the age of seven; the lateral incisor at eight; the first permanent bicuspid succeeds the temporary first molar at nine; and the second bicuspid, the second temporary molar at ten; and the cuspids are changed at the age of eleven. These are approximate ages with, of course, some considerable variation in the cases of different individuals. The second permanent molar appears at about the age of twelve, and the third molar, or wisdom tooth, at sixteen or at any time thereafter.

Bearing in mind what I have said of the appearance of the first permanent molar at the age of six, while the tooth which comes into place immediately forward of it, replacing the temporary second molar, is not due until the age of ten, and remembering the fact that any tooth in the back of the mouth has a marked disposition to move forward if there is any opportunity for such motion, it follows that if the temporary second molar is prematurely lost the six year molar moves forward into the space rightfully belonging to the second bicuspid, so that when the second bicuspid is ready to appear four years later, the room to which it is rightfully entitled has been largely appropriated by the six year molar. This leads to a crowding and irregularity of the teeth about the front of the mouth which is deplorable. Irregularity of the teeth is a thing to be regretted, not only on account of its unsightliness, but because it facilitates the inception of several diseases destructive to teeth. Nowadays instead of " irregularity " of the teeth dentists prefer the term, malocclusion. This takes cognizance of the fact that the right relations to each other of the teeth in the opposing jaws is of material consequence for the proper performance of the function of mastication.

If at the time of eruption the teeth do not come into their right relationships with each other it is desirable that the dentist's aid be sought early. There is among those who make a specialty of correcting malocclusion, orthodontists as they are called, a consensus of opinion that it is better to make teeth grow into their right positions than it is to undertake to put them there after they have been for a considerable time in wrong relations. The orthodontists also hold as cardinal doctrine that, with rare exceptions, all of the teeth should be preserved; in other words, that no teeth should be extracted "to make room," and that the dentist should not undertake to improve upon nature's normal type.

A related matter of supreme consequence is the condition of the child's throat. Throat obstructions of every kind, such as enlarged tonsils and adenoid growths, especially the latter, are a serious interference with the child's well-being, physically, mentally, and, as is now believed, morally. They often cause mouth-breathing; and with all the rest of their mischievous influence have much to do in making deformities in the face and jaws and in the positions of the teeth. Orthodontists, with other specialists, insist that children's throats should be made clear. Doing this contributes vastly to their health in many ways.

To the conditions mentioned should be added an important fact with reference to the development of teeth, applying also to development generally, — that precocity ordinarily means a poor quality of development, while tardiness in the development and eruption of teeth has usually associated with it excellent quality. It happens in a few instances that a baby is born with one or two teeth in sight, and that it follows up this characteristic of premature development in all of its dentition. Such teeth are almost invariably of poor quality and much inclined to decay. Nature's capacity for building at the time these teeth were prematurely formed was so limited that she could not do her best work. On the other hand, teeth that are tardily formed and tardily erupted are, as I have said, usually strong and resistant.

In order that we understand something of the philosophy of the good care of the teeth, it is desirable that we know something of their constitution, their make-up. The teeth are, in a sense, dermal structures; that is, like the hair and the nails, they might without much stretching of the fact be called modified skin. The mucous membrane, which lines all of the orifices of the body and is reflected upon a considerable portion of the interior chambers and passages, is but a modified skin, an internal skin, it might be called. Histologically, skin and mucous membrane are practically identical. They are each made up of epithelial cells, and the differences between skin and mucous membrane are differences made by differences of environment. The skin is exposed to the air, accustomed to friction, has ordinarily a dry surface, while the mucous membrane is more or less protected from atmospheric action and does not receive the dry friction to which the skin is accustomed. This fact is shown in a sense in the interchanged characteristics of skin and mucous membrane, if either, through any abnormality, becomes subjected to the environment of the other. We shall see a little later a significance of this skin-origin, if we may call it so, of the teeth.

The teeth are developed in an involuted pocket, or *cul-de-sac*, of mucous membrane. At first all of that which is to become tooth is made up of soft tissue so invested. Without going into the minutiae of tooth development, we may accept the fact that the hard tissues of the teeth are constructed by a process of calcification, or in other words, by the deposition of lime salts in this matrix of soft tissue which had preceded. The cells that are the actual builders of the dentine are called the ondontoblasts. The development of what is spoken of by dentists as the dentine, the bone of the tooth, begins upon the periphery of the organ of formation, and proceeds progressively from without inwards. A cross section of dentine is like the cross section of a tubular boiler. It is made up of a multitude of microscopically fine tubules having a packing of what is called the intertubular substance, and containing something which has the capacity of conveying sensation. The most powerful microscopes which have ever been made are unable to demonstrate the penetration to any considerable distance, except in rare instances, of nerve tissue into the dentinal tubules; but all who have had a sensitive cavity prepared for filling will testify that something exists in the constitution of the dentine, which has a lively capacity for conveying sensation. This construction of dentine, while it is largely completed by the time the tooth has fully erupted, attaining its place among its fellows in the jaw, continues to go on slowly through life.

That which is spoken of commonly as the nerve of the tooth is made up partly of nervous tissue, but it includes also arterial and venous capillaries for the nutrition of the parts, with connective tissue as a packing material. Inasmuch as but a portion of this substance is nerve, it is more accurate to speak of it as the pulp of the tooth. From what we have just seen, the pulp was originally as large as the completed tooth, minus the enamel, and the cementum which covers the root; and what is usually spoken of as the nerve, or as we say, the pulp, is but the remains of the formative organ, and is the main dependence of the formed tooth for its nutrition continuously through life. It grows somewhat smaller through additional calcification about the periphery. In people of advanced age the pulp becomes extremely attenuated, almost obliterated.

The enamel of the tooth begins to form at the same place where the formation of dentine commenced, and goes on progressively from within outwards, so that the construction of enamel is finished at the surface. A cross section of enamel reveals a construction of six-sided prisms of great resisting capacity when the formation is perfect. As a matter of fact this construction of enamel is imperfect in multitudes of instances. Calcification of enamel begins on the prominent parts of the teeth crowns, the cutting edges of the incisors, the points of the cuspids and bicuspids, and the eminences of the molars. In the bicuspids and molars it progresses from the eminences laterally down into the valleys, the sulci of the teeth, and there is supposed to unite so completely as to form an unbroken sheet of enamel over the entire crown. If the formation is perfect, this is what has taken place; but, as I said, in multitudes of instances, the enamel formed from these different centers fails to coalesce at what should have been the point of union, and there remains a fissure or seam of imperfect construction.

CARE OF THE TEETH

Now as we are studying the matter of preservation of the teeth, we need to get an understanding of what are the greatest dangers to which the teeth are exposed. These dangers are principally two: first, dental caries, what is popularly known as decay of the teeth; and second, diseases of the investments of the teeth, by which teeth in themselves often intrinsically good, are lost.

In the first place, with reference to dental caries, a disease of universal prevalence so far as civilized people are concerned, and familiar to every one of us. The matter of causation was studied through the lives of many generations of men without the attainment of anything like full and positive knowledge upon the subject. As in the investigation of many other things which have been for a time uncertain, knowledge has been gained step by step, until within the last quarter of a century we have come to what is practically a full understanding of what are the influences that occasion the decay of teeth.

We have seen that the hard tissues of the teeth are made up principally of salts of lime, largely the carbonate and phosphate of lime. This means that they are susceptible to the influence of chemical action that may attack constructions of salts of lime, or in other words, they are susceptible to the action of acids, and may be destroyed by such action. Indeed, a French investigator, the late Doctor E. Magitot, as the result of a good many experiments which he instituted, arrived at the conclusion that dental caries was a purely chemical solution of the lime salts of the teeth in acids. But there was a fallacy in Magitot's conclusions for the reason that in his experiments he did not duplicate conditions as they exist in the mouth. He did produce disintegration of enamel and dentine by the action of acids; but that is not dental caries as it exists under natural conditions. To grasp the whole etiology of dental caries, we need to take cognizance of the constant and practically inevitable presence of multitudes of microörganisms in the tooth environment. ·The mouth is an ideal culture chamber, — in its temperature, in its moisture, in its abundance of acceptable nutrition, and in all the environment which it provides for germ life. These microörganisms are of many varieties. For our present purpose, we may speak especially of those which have a capacity for the induction of fermentation. As you doubtless know, ordinary fermentation is inevitably dependent upon the presence and the life activities of microorganisms of certain types. Without the presence of these microörganisms, no fermentation of this kind is possible. These are truths that in their practical manifestations and demonstrations are more or less familiar to all of us, — perhaps prominently so in the fermentation or souring of certain articles of food, as for instance milk, and fruits and vegetables of various kinds. Advantage is taken of this knowledge of the function of micro-organisms in inducing fermentation of different substances, to counteract, by various expedients, the operation of microörganisms, as for instance, by heating to a germicidal temperature a substance that is to be preserved, with or without the addition of sugar or other agencies that have the quality of preserving the substances. If any food material be absolutely sterilized in its fresh and wholesome condition and then be sealed from contact with micro-organisms, its preservation, practically unchanged, is a thing accomplished for indefinite time. Familiar examples of fermentation are the fermentation of wine, of beer, of cider. As you know, there are various and successive kinds of fermentations to which such products are subject, each bringing about its own type of change.

Bear in mind that in that class of fermentations with which we are now concerned, a factor prominent in the results of fermentation is the formation of acid. This is shown by the at least partially synonymous use of the term " souring " for fermentation. We say that the apple-sauce has fermented, or has soured; and everybody understands.

Wherever life exists something is consumed, something is transformed; something which is a waste product for the organism first concerned is developed. And this waste product is often of far more consequence as a disease producer than the microörganisms themselves. In other words, in many cases it is the ptomaines that induce the disease, as it is the microörganisms that produce the ptomaines. This indirect mischief-making of the microörganisms obtains to a large extent in tooth diseases, as we shall see.

Perhaps some people still hold to the supposition that the microörganisms producing these changes, particularly the changes in the mouth, are animal parasites, that is, that they are in themselves minute animals. This is an error. Although we may sometimes jokingly speak of the " bugs " in the mouth they are not "bugs." With extremely few exceptions the disease-producing microorganisms flourishing in the mouth and in the other regions of the body are believed to be in their nature and constitution vegetable and not animal. They are a particularly simple and minute form of vegetable life, and they may be compared to some of the other low forms of vegetable life plainly apparent to the ordinary senses, such as lichens and mosses. Just as we may see patches of moss growing upon a ledge of rock, particularly in a damp place and upon a stone surface not exposed to much friction, we find that these microörganisms of the mouth have a capacity of forming among themselves colonies of millions of individuals, constituting a " plaque," and attaching or agglutinating themselves to the tooth surface, with the result that the tooth surface to which they are attached undergoes disintegration on account of their presence; just as we shall find if we detach the moss from the ledge that there are visible evidences of some disintegration of the rock surface on account of its having contributed to the support of the moss. It is an illustration of the great fact that it is impossible to get something out of nothing.

This analogy between the moss on the rock and the bacterial plaque on the tooth should be studied a little further. It is an old saying that " A rolling stone gathers no moss." This is rightly taken to be an impressive, emphasized statement of figurative truth, through the assertion of a physical fact so patent that no one could think of disputing it. The impacts and friction to which the rolling stone is subject keep it free from attachments of parasitic life, — keep its surface clean. Almost as positively as this, we can say that the tooth surface which is habitually well frictionized will be kept clear of adhesions of mischief-making microörganisms, and will not suffer from disintegration and decay. Indeed the rule applies more emphatically to the tooth than to the stone, because in the tooth the friction acts as a stimulation to the natural constructive powers to increase the strength of the resistance, and dead stone has no such powers. I shall revert to this matter later. Putting the teeth to real service in chewing food that requires earnest mastication, their proper function, is markedly for their advantage. Disuse, or little use, invites disease.

These things have been rehearsed in order to help in understanding what are the disintegrative influences upon teeth in the mouth.

Having before us these matters of tooth constitution, of the chemical nature of the teeth, of existing imperfection in the formation of the teeth, of the presence in the mouth of various fermentable substances, and also of the existence there of millions of micro-organisms capable of inducing fermentation, we have a grasp of a large part of the causation of tooth decay.

The assertion may be made that a clean tooth never decays; and this comes very near being strictly true. So far as comes to my mind it is completely and positively true, if we explain that by a clean tooth, we mean one that is materially, physically, chemically, and bacteriologically clean. Compliance with these conditions should eliminate dental caries.

Now we turn aside for a moment to make a division into two classes of all cavities occurring in teeth. You remember what I said about imperfections in the formation of the enamel of the teeth, — the pits' and fissures and seams and imperfect places in the teeth, which make interruptions in the continuity of the enamel sheet. When I was speaking of such things, I might have stated that illness, particularly of the exanthematous type, occurring in young children at the period in their life history when the teeth are undergoing the process of calcifying, often leaves its marks in the shape of grooves or a row of pits transversely upon the teeth, occasioned by nature's modified capacity for construction during the illness. These are comparable to the marks of imperfection in the formation of the finger nails, often apparent after severe illnesses in adults. It is like the flaw in the weaver's web if the shuttle does not pass as it should as the web is being advanced in the loom. We make our first great group of cavities in the teeth include those cavities which have their initiation in the fissures of original imperfect formation. They come very largely upon what are called the grinding surfaces of the molars and in the valleys of the bicuspids. Here the process of decay is invited and facilitated in ways which we are about to see. We put in our second group of cavities those which are formed upon surfaces of teeth where the original construction involved no imperfection. In this second class of cavities, we shall find almost invariably a disadvantage of environment which made the attainment of any good degree of cleanliness a much more difficult thing than in the case of surfaces that are freely exposed to friction. Practically speaking a tooth surface receiving from mastication or any other circumstance a good deal of friction is thereby exempted from an attack of caries.

Now, bearing in mind these circumstances of unfavorable environment, of untidiness, of accumulation of debris of food, of oral fluids little moved or changed and really stagnated, we are prepared to come back to our theory of causation of disintegration of teeth by decay.

This debris accumulated around the teeth is acceptable and congenial pabulum for multitudes of microörganisms which flourish there, and as a result of their life history produce acids. Just as we have seen the souring of milk from the presence of an acid-producing microorganism, we may see a like process taking place in the mouth with like results; and the acid thus formed directly upon those surfaces of the teeth less exposed to friction begins a process of disintegration of enamel which is the first step in the formation of cavities which come upon tooth surfaces where there was no original defective formation. This means that cavities of what we are calling the second class come in between the teeth especially if there are places in which food habitually lodges and is permitted to remain. Such cavities come also at the necks of teeth, at the margin of the gums, if there is not tidiness and care in the removal of the remains of food. They are especially likely to come about the third molar or wisdom tooth on account of the general unfavorableness of the environment. Often these teeth are not fully erupted. They may remain for years only partially through, not yet occupying their right places, with possibly a flap of the gum partially overlapping them and making a pocket for the retention of particles of food and other debris. The cheek often lies in close apposition with the surface of the tooth, and in all particulars the environment is most unfavorable. To this is often added inefficiency in the means of cleaning, when the tooth brush is not made to reach so far back as these teeth. This is very largely the explanation of the popular idea that the wisdom tooth is the poorest tooth in the mouth. As a matter of fact, being formed last, when the tooth-building powers of the system are at their best, the wisdom tooth is frequently very well constituted; but it is the unfortunate victim of its surroundings. In numerous instances it is more sinned against than sinning.

After the action of the product of microörganisms, and note that I say the action of the product of microörganisms, because no microörganism in itself has any capacity to attack and disintegrate tooth substance, and remembering the physical and chemical make-up of enamel and dentine, we are prepared to see that the conjoined action of micro-organisms and acid constitute the active agencies in the production of decay. As a matter of fact, no microörganism is so small as to be able to penetrate into the sound dentine. They are all too large to be accommodated within the diameter of the dentinal tubule. When the dentine has undergone softening by the acid action, the microörganisms are able to penetrate the tubules, and do penetrate them and carry on the process of fermentation with the result of acid formation in the cavity of decay. Thus it is that the more organisms, the more formation of acid, the more acid formation, the more disintegration of lime salts, the more softening of the dentinal tubules, the more penetration of organisms within the tubules, all together pushing on the process of disintegration and decay.

Now, leaving this, let us consider the other great class of oral diseases whose action occasions the loss of many good teeth, namely, disease of the investments of the teeth, disease of the gums, disease of the bony sockets of the teeth. This is often spoken of as recession of the gums, spongy gums, elongation of the teeth, loosening of the teeth, or by other such names. There are various popular names for it, and various other names used by dentists. A designation a good deal used is "Riggs' disease." This term is in recognition of the part which the late Dr. John M. Riggs, of Hartford, took about forty-five years ago in pointing out a considerable share of its true pathology. It is called by dentists *pyorrhoea alveolaris*, which means literally, a flow of pus from the alveolus, that is, from the tooth socket. It is spoken of sometimes as *interstitial gingivitis*, which signifies inflammation within the substance of the gums, sometimes as *phagedenic percementitis*, which means a wasting inflammation about the roots. It is an affection whose causation, although partially understood for a good many years, has not been thoroughly comprehended until very recently; and it is no doubt true that we have not yet come to understand all that is to be learned and that we ought to know about this disease.

Dr. Riggs' own theory of it was that it was very largely due to accumulations of foreign substances, such as are popularly spoken of as tartar, about the teeth. This formation is ordinarily greatest upon those tooth surfaces situated opposite to the openings of the ducts which bring saliva into the mouth, or in other words upon the lingual aspect of the lower front teeth and the buccal side of the upper molars.

The saliva may hold in suspension salts of lime chemically resembling the salts of lime which constitute a large part of the teeth. These salts are likely to be deposited upon any hard stationary surface which may be in their way. The deposit of tartar ordinarily begins at the margin of the gum in positions not well exposed to friction, and gradually increases, extending itself upon the exposed portion of the crown of the tooth and insinuating itself under the margin of the gum upon the root, occasioning irritation and extending farther and farther, until it loosens the attachment of the gum to the tooth, induces a marked congestion and chronic inflammation of the soft tissues with morbific discharges, including, in deep-seated cases, the constant production of pus. There also appears in these deep-seated cases some loss of vitality of the thin margin of the bony socket of the tooth, the alveolus; and this may progress in connection with the other recession and may go on until nearly or quite all of the socket has vanished. The tooth becomes extremely loose, and either falls out of itself, or becomes so troublesome that it is purposely removed.

It has been the theory of our English professional friends that in this disease, the primary disturbance was in the bony tissue of the margin of the socket; and that the other manifestations, including the deposit of calculus, were to be classed among consequences rather than causes of the disease. I have no doubt that there is a very small percentage of cases in which this is true, cases of caries and necrosis of bone and of mercurialization; but the general truth of our own ideas about it appears to be supported by the undenied fact that, practically speaking, the disease always vanishes promptly when the teeth with their attached deposits are removed.

Another theory with reference to the cause of this affection is the microörganic theory. Without any manner of doubt, there are numerous cases in which microorganisms do have a part in carrying forward the affection. This would seem to be proved by the fact that in numbers of cases the use of autogenous vaccines prepared from cultures from the individual mouths, or even stock vaccines of microörganisms of types having much to do in causing suppuration, is often followed by most gratifying results in mitigating, if not curing, the disease.

Very recent discoveries appear to show in a large proportion of these cases the presence of pus-producing parasites, animal in their nature, which may be killed by a specific germicide. From limited experience the claim is made that this treatment in connection with the proper instrumentation goes far toward relieving the trouble.

Another causative factor in this affection is believed to be inefficiency, incompleteness or tardiness in the elimination of waste products, especially through the alimentary canal, and the kidneys. Habitual costiveness, the undue retention within the system of waste material which should have been rejected, without doubt leads in some cases to a vicarious elimination in which the mouth suffers. A similar statement may be made about the failure of the kidneys to carry out of the system those wastes which it is their proper function to excrete.

One thing that is absolutely sure about this disease when it has once become deeply established is that it can never cure itself or come to an end spontaneously, with anything short of the loss of the teeth. Another sure thing is that in any treatment of the trouble which the dentist institutes there can be no real success unless that treatment includes the thorough removal of all concretions from the surfaces of the teeth, and especially and emphatically from those surfaces of the teeth that are beneath the gum.

There are most important relationships between these mouth diseases and systemic diseases of a variety of types. In many cases the mouth disease stands in a causative relation to the other disease; but those are things which we cannot include in this study now.

One other general fact should be brought into the reckoning; and that is that the habitual chemical quality of the oral fluids has a good deal to do with this matter of caries and also of deposits upon the teeth. It is believed that the chemical condition of the oral fluids is intended to be slightly alkaline. It should at least be neutral. If it is slightly alkaline there are therein advantages. One of these is that the food in the process of mastication and insalivation is saturated with a fluid somewhat alkaline and is thereby the better prepared for stomach digestion, a process carried on largely by the gastric juice, which has marked acidity as one of its characteristics. A further advantage, and one of great practical consequence in connection with our present study, is that this alkalinity gives protection for the teeth from the action of acids to which they are frequently exposed, such as, for instance, the acids of condiments and of many fruits, like apples, peaches, oranges, grapes, strawberries, etc. Whenever there is produced by these things the sensation of the teeth being " set on edge " the explanation lies in the superficial corrosion and irritation by the acid.

The dentist often sees, particularly in the case of young girls who are not fully developed, and are perhaps overworking in school, or combining with their work too great devotion to society, with late hours, and making various mischievous inclusions in their diet, mouths that show unmistakably the habitual presence of acidity. Associated with that acidity are almost inevitably to be found the ravages of extensive decay, extreme sensitiveness, and an entire absence of calcareous deposits or tartar. In such a case more can be done for the well-being of the teeth by eliminating the unhygienic factors in the patient's life and by building up the general health, getting nature's functions established, maintaining a proper regimen in all particulars, and especially by antagonizing the acid condition, than can possibly be accomplished by the dentist in his operations of filling cavities alone.

More rarely there may be such extreme alkalinity of the oral fluids, such a superabundance of lime salts held in suspension, that there become attached to the teeth great quantities of calcic concretions from which it is extremely difficult to keep them free. These are in no way a menace to the tooth structure itself. They do not cause decay; but their influence is likely to be in the direction of causing Riggs' disease. In antagonizing hyperalkalinity we do not know how to do directly and safely very much with chemical agents, for the reason that the constitution of calcareous concretions is chemically so similar to the constitution of the teeth themselves that whatever is capable of attacking one is likely to attack the other.

Now, without following this any further, we have compassed, I am sure, an understanding of what agencies are very powerful workers against the well-being of the teeth, and have had at least suggestions as to what are helpful measures to use in their preservation.

All of these considerations point to the fact that the intelligent use of agencies for maintaining a good degree of cleanliness of the teeth is of great consequence in attaining freedom from disease, and in antagonizing the influences that tend to the disintegration and loss of the teeth. The faithful and intelligent use of a brush of proper quality, not too hard and not too soft, supplemented by such dentifrices and mouth washes as may be useful in particular cases (not the same for all people), with the use of silk drawn between the teeth to cleanse the surfaces most in need of cleaning and most susceptible to decay, are our main reliances. When conveniently possible they should be used after eating, particularly after the last meal of the day. The most important time is before retiring at night. If the teeth may not be brushed after some of the meals the thorough rinsing of the mouth may be helpful.

To this care should be added, of course, if needed, the counteracting or antagonizing, or better still, the prevention of acid conditions.

In the antagonizing of acid we have four principal agents, all of which are useful in various degrees. The first of these is prepared chalk which chemically neutralizes acid. It constitutes the basis of most of the good dentifrices. A second means of locally antagonizing acid in the mouth is bicarbonate of soda. There are some objections alleged to the use of this remedy; but I believe that they are theoretical rather than practical. As much sodium bicarbonate as can be held upon a dime, dissolved in a small glass of warm water and used in rinsing the mouth, is one of the helps in antagonizing acidity. Another good antacid is lime water. Lime is soluble in water only to a very slight extent; and it may be very conveniently prepared for use by first satisfying its affinity for water, or in other words slaking it. For this there should be used a clean piece of board, or something which will not be broken by the sudden development of heat when the lime and water are brought together. Put the mixture in a bottle, and fill with water, and you will always have conveniently at hand a saturated solution of lime. This may be diluted somewhat with plain water, but ordinarily need not be much diluted. If made not disagreeably strong, it may be used freely as a mouth wash. It may also be used advantageously as an addition to milk, to facilitate its digestibility and avoid curds in the stomach and prevent gastric acidity.

A fourth and most effective agency for antagonizing acidity is milk of magnesia. This is not a thing to be used in brushing and cleaning the teeth; but its use should follow the cleaning agencies, particularly at night, by taking a small teaspoonful of the milk of magnesia into the mouth, and with the tongue and cheeks smearing it over the teeth. In this way its influence is very persistent and efficient.

The teeth ordinarily decay more during the quiescence of the mouth at night than they do during the day; and this use of magnesia brings the helpful agency into service at the time when it can do the most good.

To speak a little more about dentifrices — they are almost without exception innocent and more or less effective. Some are much better than others; but there is little occasion for incorporating in them anything injurious; and those that are produced and sold by reputable pharmacists are almost invariably free from any harmful quality. The street fakir who works a transformation from the unsightliness of the teeth of the gamin probably uses a preparation containing alum or some kind of acid; but such agencies are not likely to be used by intelligent people. Some of the newer proprietary preparations whose well chosen ingredients are declared, so combine germicidal influence with the right abrasive quality and a capacity for antagonizing acids as to make them superior preparations. I suppose that in this place I ought not to make mention of any particular preparation; but I have confidence in the general beneficial influence of the better specimens of the class that I have in mind, not only for their good effect upon the teeth, but as having much influence in lessening the pathogenic microörganisms of the mouth and throat, and so contributing materially to the user's well-being in other ways. Special dentifrices and mouth washes for individual needs should be prescribed or provided by the dentist.

The manner of using the brush in order that good and not harm may result should be mentioned. Occasionally a person with more zeal than discretion, using a stiff brush and a coarse powder with a crosswise motion of the brush over the necks of the teeth, does make mischief. The margin of the gum is fretted and forced back, the softer portion of the tooth above or below the enamel border is exposed, and may be materially worn so as to constitute a V-shaped groove, markedly for the tooth's disadvantage. The right way to use the brush is to place it upon the gum and with a half-rotary motion bring it perpendicularly upward upon the lower teeth, downward on the upper teeth, in such a way as to avoid this danger of mischief which has just been described as possible in the crosswise motion. With this motion of the brush, not only is no harm likely to come to the soft tissues, but the cleansing of the teeth will be much more efficient through the passing of the bristles of the rightly trimmed toothbrush between the teeth, than could possibly be the case if the crosswise motion were used. The bristles of the brush should not be set together too compactly, and they may well be trimmed so as to give the brush a serrated face.

Of course, when we are considering the means of preserving the natural teeth we have to include the dentist's services. In the arrest of dental decay by the process of filling, in antagonizing disease of the investments of the teeth through the removal of foreign deposits, and in the treatment of numerous pathological conditions as they arise in and about the teeth and mouth the dentist's services are for the average individual absolutely indispensable. No class of men would be more glad to have teeth cease to need repairing than would dentists, just as no other class of men would be so glad to have humanity cease to suffer from general diseases as would physicians. And there is a way of practicing dentistry which is capable, and has been proved to be capable, of setting aside a large part of the ills to which teeth are heir. This is a system which is spoken of as prophylaxis, which comes from a Greek word which signifies prevention. We are told that in China there is a practice of medicine through which the patient pays to his medical adviser a salary, and this salary goes on so long as the patient remains well. The instant the patient becomes ill the salary stops and stays stopped until the patient is restored to health. Dental prophylaxis has resemblance to this. The dentist is paid for preventing dental caries and pyorrhoea alveolaris, not for repairing or attempting to repair the mischief after it has been done. As sometimes pursued, this system gives the dentist an annual salary. The dentist on his part, insists on having an opportunity to give the teeth a thorough cleansing and scrubbing once a month regularly. This process commenced in children and persistently followed up, aided by the intelligent coöperation of the patients in maintaining cleanliness, does result in the prevention of a very large number of decay cavities of our second class, those upon the surfaces where there was originally perfection of formation. You will be the better prepared to believe this by going back to the fact, stated earlier, that the teeth are in a sense modified dermal structures, with many of the characteristics of such structures. One of these characteristics of especial consequence in the present connection is the effect of friction, of a good deal of friction often repeated. When this comes upon the skin it induces a thickening and hardening, intended by nature for self-defence, like the callosity in the hand of the man who does rough work, and the thickening of the skin on the bottom of the feet.

If the dentist has the opportunity to begin the application of this system with a stick and pumice stone on all of the tooth surfaces of a young child, and keeps up this process faithfully, there is developed in the tooth tissue, greatly increased hardness and resistive capacity. Were people to adopt this system, and were the cavities consequent upon imperfection in formation cut out and filled early there would be practically almost no more occasion for filling of teeth. Pyorrhoeal conditions would be altogether prevented, and there would be maintained constantly a dental and oral health beautiful to see and delightful to experience. The visit to the dentist would lose its terrors; and the patient would go to the dental office with the same equanimity as if the visit were a visit to the manicure.

The other things which I wish to say have regard to popular ideas more or less generally held. One of these is that sweet things occasion a great deal of trouble with teeth. This is very largely an error. Sugar, so long as it remains sugar, is absolutely incapable of harmfully influencing sound tooth tissue. When not taken in excess and at unsuitable times and if taken in a way so as to form legitimately a part of the diet to be digested with other food, sugar is not only harmless, but provides material needed for the nutrition of the body and the maintenance of its temperature. The mischief from sweets comes through their supplying a substance that is capable of comparatively ready fermentation in the mouth and in the stomach. They may be taken in such quantities as to impair the digestion, and to lead to a decided acidity which, if not directly developed in the mouth, is conveyed from the stomach to the marked disadvantage of the teeth. But the accusation which dentists very frequently hear parents bring against children, that the decay of their teeth, and their toothaches are due to the use of sweets, is in most instances injustice.

Another idea is that the period of gestation and lactation in women is a time fraught with peculiar danger to the teeth. The popular idea, popularly expressed, is that " every child costs its mother a tooth." There is some foundation for this belief. The explanation is partly in the extra demand upon the mother's system in the nourishment of the new being during the pregnancy; but probably to a greater extent the harm to the teeth comes as a consequence of the derangement of the mother's system. Not rarely during pregnancy there is disturbance of digestion as manifest in the morning sickness. The vomiting of pregnancy has associated with it marked acidity. This prevailing acidity is largely the explanation of the lesions which take place in teeth during gestation. In the light of all of the facts presented, there appears the logical deduction that at this period there should be especial care in the use of means to antagonize acid conditions.

Another idea which dentists hear expressed almost constantly is that medicines are great mischief-makers for teeth. "I always had good teeth until I had a fit of sickness, and then the doctors gave me so many medicines that my teeth were ruined." This is usually rank injustice to the physician; and the dentist should be earnest in correcting the patient's erroneous beliefs. Ordinarily the troubles with the teeth are due to the illness and conditions associated with the illness, and not to the medicines. Almost all medicines as now used are harmless to teeth; but there are a few that may injure teeth or their investments. When one has included acids, salts from which acids may be liberated, some of the iron preparations and the mercurials, the latter particularly when pushed to the extent of producing salivation, the list is nearly complete.

There are cases, particularly of children, in which it is desirable to provide the system with special nutrition for the teeth. An established fact in this connection is that if lime salts are to be supplied in the diet for the good development of the teeth and the bones, they should be the lime salts which are prepared by nature rather than in the chemist's laboratory. Synthetically produced lime salts are not assimilated and appropriated into the body; they pass out very largely as they entered; but the lime salts which nature produces, the lime salts in eggs, in meat, in milk and in cereals, are in the shape that nature can assimilate, and appropriate to the nutrition of the tissues which are formed of such materials. If we are to administer special lime salts it is believed that the lactophosphate, really prepared from milk, is among the most advantageous.

The maintenance of good systemic health, good digestion, good assimilation, good nutrition, good elimination of waste, the proper performance of function generally, has much to do with the health of the mouth and exemption from dental and oral diseases.

PRINTED AT
THE HARVARD UNIVERSITY PRESS
CAMBRIDGE, MASS., U.S.A.